Pilates
Walk

Tips, Techniques, and Exercises
for a Healthy Stride

Aliesa George, PMA-CPT

Pilates-Walk™

Tips, Techniques, and Exercises for a Healthy Stride

Aliesa George, PMA-CPT

Published by Centerworks® Pilates LLC
520 S. Holland, Suite 201-203, Wichita, KS 67209 USA
www.Centerworks.com

Printed in the United States of America

ISBN: 978-0-9889468-3-5

Library of Congress Control Number: 2016916621

SPECIAL THANKS AND ACKNOWLEDGEMENTS

This Pilates-Walk™ health improvement project has been 20 years in the making! I'd like to thank the thousands of clients I've had the privilege to work with over the past twenty plus years, as we've used Pilates training as a tool to improve whole-body health and worked together to develop healthier movement habits.

Walking is something we take for granted when our body feels great. But it's something that we find painful and life-altering when it hurts to walk, or if we can't walk due to an injury or accident. Whether it's in our foot, knee, hip, back, shoulder, or neck, when pain affects our ability to move around for daily life activities, there's not even the thought of walking for exercise!

Even before I started teaching Pilates, I helped clients in the health club learn to walk more efficiently to get better results from their workouts. For the past 22 years, I have taught Pilates and foot fitness workshops, worked with both clients and teachers in the studio, and have done various other sports and physical activities which form, posture, and gait were key elements. It has become clear to me that there is so much to be gained from teaching people how to get the most out of an essential activity that they do countless times a day: walking. Piece by piece, as I've had the privilege to work with each and every one of my clients, this Pilates-Walk™ training system has been born.

Special thanks to my mentors and Pilates teachers:

David Mooney, my first Pilates teacher, who taught me the value of breaking down exercises and building them back up to deepen the mind-body connection and really help find and feel the right muscles working.

Romana Krayzanowska, who mentored my initial Pilates certification program – for showing the value of working the body with rhythm and pacing. She gave me an understanding of the systematic order of exercises in the Pilates workout program as well as the multiple progressive levels that continuously challenge and condition the body. My experience as her student was truly enlightening; it has increased my understanding of the value of the Pilates method for improving whole-body health and has helped me develop safe and effective training programs.

And finally, Dianne Miller, who is not only a mentor, but dear friend, who has shared her insights for improving functional movement and developing better body mechanics for Pilates and life. I am so lucky that our paths have crossed in this lifetime! Everything I have learned from you has helped me become a better teacher, and teacher-trainer, and has truly made the difference in my ability to see and correct clients to help them connect mind, body, and spirit and enjoy lasting results from their Pilates training programs.

I cherish every second of time I've had learning more about Pilates and the body. And I absolutely love how Pilates principles transfer to everyday life, and can be so easily practiced to improve whole-body health and wellness thru walking.

Thank you for letting me share my passion for Pilates-Walk™ with YOU!

Aliesa George

TABLE OF CONTENTS

DISCLAIMER

Not all exercises are suitable for everyone. Please consult with your doctor before beginning this or any exercise program to ensure your safety and reduce the risk of injury. The instructions presented herein are in no way intended as a substitute for medical counseling. If you have had a joint replacement, or if you have osteoporosis, are recovering from an injury or accident, or have any other special medical conditions, follow all exercise guidelines and precautions as outlined by your physician.

My Mission, and the Pilates-Walk™ goal is to give you lots of helpful information and exercise tips so that you can find and use the right muscles when you walk.

Walking is one of the best whole-body wellness activities (*when your form is good*). But with poor posture and bad body mechanics even a leisurely stroll can leave you feeling worse instead of better.

To help you maximize the benefits of your walking technique, I'm going to share with you some simple common-sense strategies and exercises that I've found helpful for myself and my Pilates clients to fine-tune their form to get more of the right muscles working to walk well.

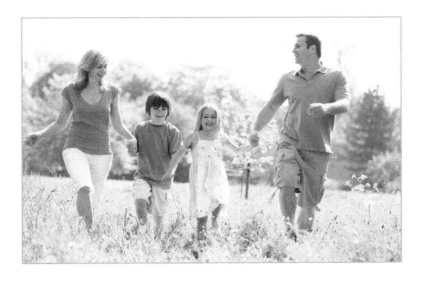

Everybody walks! Whether walking is a part of your workout routine, or just something you to do get you from one place to the next, how your body is moving directly relates to how it feels. Poor posture and movement habits can only lead to aches, pains, and injuries. Practicing healthy movement habits will lead you down the road to better health!

This book is designed to be a handbook, and guide to help you become more aware of your current walking habits, and help you tweak your technique for better form and function.

The more efficient your gait, the better your stride; the better your stride, the more you use the correct muscles to move. Walking with good body alignment will help keep you strong, fit, flexible, and – most importantly – injury-free.

Whether you're walking down the block, or doing marathons, Pilates-Walk™ Movement Strategies can help you feel well and be well.

So don't just sit there and read this book... Get up, start moving, and practice the exercises! Improving your body awareness and re-training your walking habits to be healthier will only happen when you take action with a focus on your form and function.

Be Well and Enjoy Your Pilates-Walk Workouts!

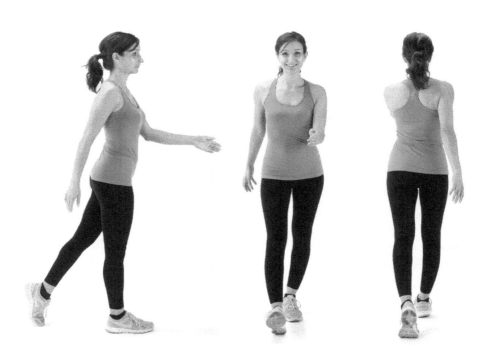

Chapter 1

What Is Pilates?

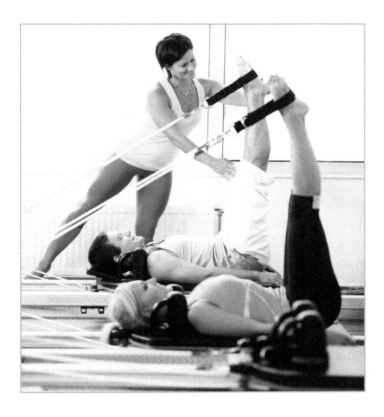

Pilates has been around since the early 1920's. This fabulous exercise system has been used for everything from rehabilitation to training professional athletes.

Regardless of who you are, or your current fitness level, there is always an appropriate place to start improving your health with Pilates.

Pilates develops both strength and flexibility. The focus is teaching you how to use your body well – finding all the right muscles so that your body is well-supported, well-balanced, and you have the strength, flexibility, and stamina to do everyday movements and tasks (*in addition to the activities you enjoy*) with zest and ease.

I have been blessed to witness the transformational health benefits of Pilates training in my own body, and have been sharing my passion for Pilates with my clients now for more than twenty years.

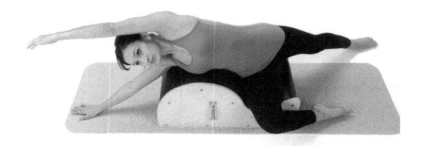

Some clients get started because they have back or shoulder problems; other people are triathletes or dancers who are healthy and fit and want to stay in shape for peak performance. Others have had injuries – sick and tired of living with chronic aches and pains – they are ready to take control of their health and take action to feel better.

Not everyone is actually looking for ways to be more efficient with what they're doing. The primary goal is to feel good and be healthy. Efficiency is a valuable result of adopting healthy movement habits. The more precise and confident you are in your movement, not only will you be able to do things more quickly, but you may find yourself tackling tasks you had previously avoided. As a walk to the mailbox becomes easier, parking in a distant space at the mall doesn't seem so daunting. As knee pain decreases or disappears, those two flights of stairs at the office can become a morning habit that replaces the elevator. Better movement habits not only improve health, but also enrich the quality of your life by enhancing your ability to do all of your current tasks while making you feel capable and confident enough to try new things!

Almost everyone at some point in life has experienced at least one minor injury or accident. What might seem like an insignificant moment in time, can actually be a life-altering event that causes our muscles to get a little bit out of balance. We start feeling better and assume that everything is ok, but those muscle imbalances are still in our system. This is a part of the reason why it's so easy to re-injure something after you've had a problem.

One of the biggest benefits of Pilates training is that it improves body awareness and identifies your muscle weaknesses and imbalances. The goal with every workout is to bring your body into balance for optimal function.

Pilates is about whole-body health, and walking is one of the most wonderful whole-body aerobic activities that you can do. If you take what you know about your body, and what you learn about healthy movement habits with Pilates training, then apply it to your walking, the result is a fantastic whole-body health workout.

Why do Pilates? You can do Pilates for a lifetime and never stop learning new things about how to use your body well. Specialized equipment and a series of Matwork exercise are the basic tools of the Pilates system. There are well over 500 different Pilates exercises utilizing the Reformer, the Trapeze Table (or Cadillac), the Pilates Ladder Barrel, Small Barrels, Chairs, Mat, and other small equipment.

Regardless of your age or current fitness level, there is an appropriate place to start. Every body can do Pilates. It's fun, challenging, effective, and noticeable improvements happen quickly with the right Pilates exercises in your weekly workout program.

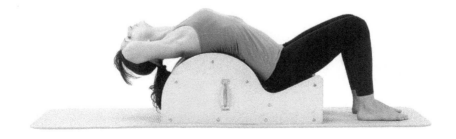

But here's the secret… Everything that you learn from Pilates applies to everything else that you do in life.

Whether you are participating in other fitness activities (*swimming, biking, running, lifting weights, playing sports*) or just daily living (*getting around in the house, standing up, sitting down, climbing stairs*), the muscles you use and the way you move should be exactly the same to stay healthy. The healthy movement habits you develop with exercise and Pilates should transfer to everything else you do in life to keep you as healthy and fit as possible.

If you have never experienced a "real" Pilates workout, that's ok (*I highly recommend you check it out with a well-qualified Pilate's teacher*). With Pilates-Walk™ training, we will take Pilates-based movement principles and apply them to easy exercises you can practice at home – no equipment needed. We will also discover helpful things to focus on while you're walking to improve your technique. Pilates experience is definitely helpful, but not required for you to get great benefits from what you'll be learning in this book.

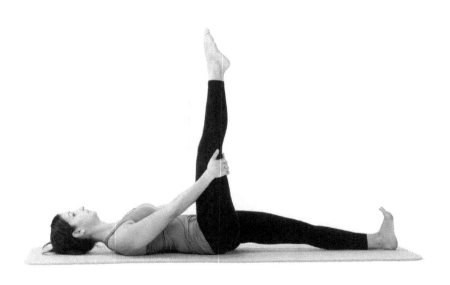

Chapter 2

The Benefits of Developing Healthy Walking Habits

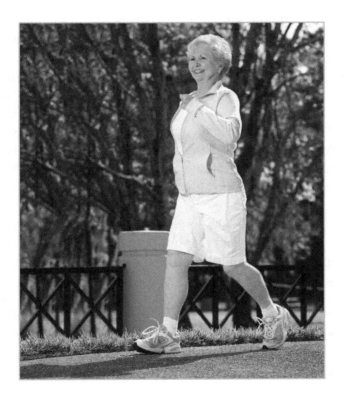

Walking is a great whole-body workout. If you think about it, when you walk, every muscle in your body is working towards making you stronger and healthier.

Done well, walking is one of the best exercises for health and wellness. Do it incorrectly or with bad muscle habits, and you're training your stronger muscles to get stronger while your weaker muscles grow weaker.

A lot of brain power is required to pay attention to your body while you're moving! Do you typically tune-in or tune-out to what your body is doing during your workouts?

The secret to developing healthy movement habits is to pay attention and be aware of how you're moving and what's working so you can make adjustments, self-correct, and fine-tune your technique to maximize the benefits from your workouts, not only when you're walking, but all the time! By paying attention to what your body is doing and focusing a little attention on your arms, your legs, your middle, your hips, your spine, your shoulders, your feet (*every piece and part of the body*), you'll discover better ways to use all of your muscles as efficiently as possible when you're moving.

With the Pilates-Walk™ system, you're going to discover new things to pay attention to for better walking technique, as well as learn simple pre-walking, or supplemental training exercises to help develop the strength and flexibility you need for healthier movement habits to walk well.

This information and these simple Pilates-Walk™ exercises will help increase your body awareness for how all your parts and pieces are put together, and how to integrate healthy movement habits into your walking workouts to be super-efficient when you're moving.

One of the many benefits of Pilates is better core strength. What better time to practice using your abdominals for support than when you're walking! In addition to a strong core, walking requires good hip strength and mobility. Lastly, without some "flipper-action" with the ankles, arches and toes, we'd just be standing still instead of moving forward.

During the process of learning some new tips and movement strategies with Pilates-Walk principles, you're going to starting finding and feeling new parts of your body working to support you better. Then we are going to incorporate these concepts and improved movement support into your walking technique. Getting started, it may feel like you've never walked a day in your life, but with practice you'll be amazed at the difference your new Pilates-Walk™ movement habits will make.

What are the benefits of walking? And why is it important to pay attention to how you are walking?

Everybody walks. Some people walk to relieve stress, sleep better, feel better, to check out the scenery, or just get outside to enjoy the fresh air. In our daily lives, we have to be able to walk from the bed to the bathroom, from the car into the office and numerous other places. Walking is not only a fitness activity to improve your health, but a necessary every day activity to get us from point A to point B.

Walking can help you look better and feel better about yourself. It can improve your heart and lung strength. Walking is a cross-patterning exercise that helps your brain. By swinging your arms and legs in opposition, walking can help improve your brain function to think better. By practicing good breathing habits while you walk (*bringing air up and down the full length of your spine*) you can maintain good posture which helps circulate cerebral spinal fluid up and down the spinal column. Feed the brain and keep it healthy. There are a million good reasons to learn how to walk well!

Walking can also help reduce or eliminate back pain. I was born with back issues, so I've had to work hard my whole life to stay active and strong enough to avoid having my back "go out," and ending up with aggravating pain. The stronger your muscles are to support good gait, the better your back is going to feel.

Walking is also one of the activities recommended for people with osteoporosis. Building bone density and doing activities where you have a little bit of impact is important to keep your bones strong, especially as we age. Poor posture and body mechanics aren't going to give you the benefits you need from walking to really help build strong bones. Good posture and body mechanics (*getting a good swing of the leg from the hip, un-leveling of the pelvis, and proper rotation of the spine*) can help provide some of the impact and movement needed to help keep your bones strong and healthy.

Think of walking as a moving meditation. Learn to enjoy complete control of both your mind and body. Develop coordination, breathing and proper body mechanics as part of good Pilates-Walking technique.

My hope is that you will discover, though your Pilates-Walk workouts how beneficial healthy movement habits are to keep you feeling great. And that this will inspire you to practice these exercises and concepts throughout your day, to help better support your body to stay healthy and fit. Do you know your goals and personal reasons for wanting to improve your walking technique?

Chapter 3

Body Awareness

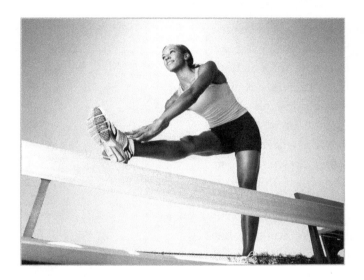

Improving your mind/body awareness is key to deepening the connection between what your body is doing and how your brain is helping to direct your movements.

I am going to share with you some targeted Pilates training tips and preparatory exercises to learn how to walk well. Your goal is to practice the prep exercises, and then try executing the movements during your Pilates-Walk workouts. Be sure to listen to your body and pay attention how things feel. Always work at a level that is appropriate for your body and current fitness level.

Pilates requires a mind/body connection. Ideally, your brain should pay attention to every movement you make from your head to your toes.

If you are not used to thinking about your whole body while it is moving, it can be a little overwhelming. So please don't get frustrated and say, "*Ahh! I can't do it all at once.*" Please know this feeling is completely normal! Everybody feels like this when they get started changing their habits. If your brain understands what I am asking you to do, that is the most important thing, because you will then be able to take what you're learning and practice in the coming weeks and months ahead.

And there's a pretty good chance your brain might be on overload with all this new information. Trying these exercise is like learning how to ride a bike. Who got on their bike the first time – without training wheels – and went whizzing down the road without falling over? Nobody!

Hopefully you're not going to fall over while you're walking but learning how to walk well and changing some of your habits is going to be similar to learning how to ride a bike. You may feel off-balance, and some of the exercise my feel strange in the beginning, but with time and repetition everything will get easier and you will get stronger and more efficient with your walking technique.

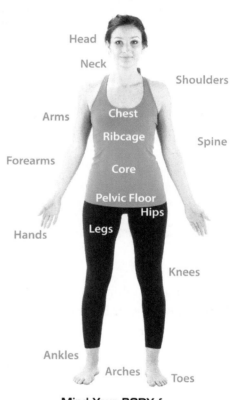

Head
Neck
Shoulders
Arms
Chest
Ribcage
Spine
Forearms
Core
Pelvic Floor
Hips
Hands
Legs
Knees
Ankles
Arches
Toes

Mind Your BODY for Healthy Movement Habits

Chapter 4

Posture

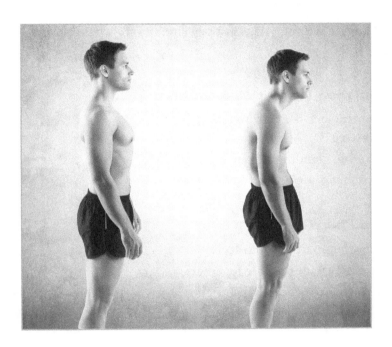

Proper posture is an essential starting point. The better your posture is while you walk, the more efficiently you will use your muscles. But if you're not aware of what you're doing when you're standing still, it becomes even more complicated when you're moving! How can you ever expect to know if you're doing things right or wrong when you're walking, if you're not aware of what you're doing when you're standing still?

Before you can make a change, you must first identify your current habits. You can evaluate your own standing posture by answering the questions that follow in this chapter. And another great evaluation tool is my quick Posture Self-Assessment Quiz, available online at www.centerworks.com.

Pilates-Walk™ Practice Exercise – Standing Posture

Note: It might be good to stand in front of a full-length mirror for this practice exercise. Stand like you would normally stand when you are not really paying much attention to your posture.

Don't change anything yet…. just pay attention to what you see, what you feel, and what you notice .

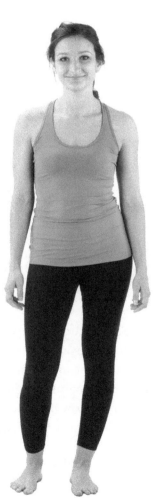

Assess Your Weight Distribution:

- Do you feel like your weight is even on both legs?
- Are you standing on one leg or both?
- Is one hip sticking off to the side?

Assess Your Feet and Legs:

- How far apart are your feet?
- Are they wide or close together?
- Are your toes pointing straight ahead?
- Can you feel if your knees are locked? Or are your knees a little bit soft? Or is one locked and one soft?

If your knees are locked, do you have knee problems or knee pain? Locked knees and knee pain tend to go together. A soft bend in the knee is going to reduce pain and problems with your knees. That small bend is also going to help strengthen the hamstring muscles along the back of your thighs.

Assess Your Torso:

- Is your belly hanging out or pulled up and in?
- Are your shoulders tense or hiked up around your ears?
- Is one shoulder higher than the other?
- Do your neck and shoulders feel relaxed?

Assess Your Head:

This is a tough one to feel. Standing in front of a mirror or having a buddy can be helpful. Getting the head stacked on the shoulders for good posture can be difficult. Even the model in this book found it to be a challenge! (*In her best posture position, the ears are still a bit in front of her shoulders*). For all of us, there's always room for improvement!

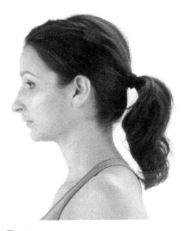

- If your ears are over your shoulders, your head is in good alignment.
- If your ears are in front of, or behind your shoulders, your head is not in alignment and there will be more tension in your neck and shoulders.

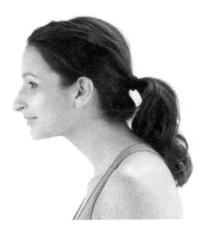

Head and Neck Posture

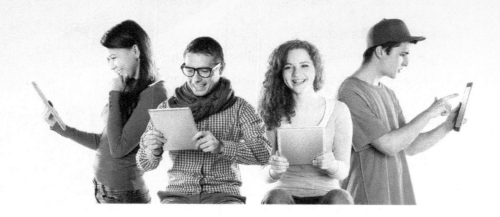

Most of us work on computers enough that we tend to jut our heads forward. It's a really bad habit. There is even a term for this forward head posture. It's called *"tech neck."*

Studies have shown, that when your spine is in neutral position, the head weighs about 10-12 pounds. At 15 degrees forward the head weighs approximately 27 pounds. At 45 degrees, it's 49 pounds, and at 60 degrees, it's 60 pounds! The problem here is, the more forward the head falls, the more gravity wins, creating more tension, not just in the neck, but throughout the entire body.

It's not just the computer – cell phones, texting, and the popularity of a digital lifestyle is making it even worse. As a result, younger people are developing the posture habits of what we used to consider the posture of *"a little old lady."*

Ultimately, you can't really *"fix"* your forward head posture, without starting with your feet and working your way up.

Our goal is to use our muscles to fight gravity so that we can stay up upright, nice and tall, young or old!

Now that you're a little more aware of your current, everyday standing posture habits, let's make some adjustments to start improving your tall posture.

Training Tips to Improve Standing Posture:

Stand with your feet as close together as you are comfortable – the closer the better. If you have knock-knees and your knees get tangled up, your feet will be slightly farther apart. If you can get your thighs all the way together, do it. Be sure both feet are pointing straight ahead.

With your legs together, hopefully you can start to feel your inner thigh muscles working. Your inner thigh muscles are important for balance. As we get older, we tend to stand with our feet wider and wider apart which means, the inner thighs don't have to work like they should and get weaker. Then, when we need them to help us balance, we don't have the support that we need, and the fear of falling increases.

Right now, even if you need to hold on to something for balance while you practice standing with your legs together, do it! You need to get stronger in this position for a healthy stride.

It's important to realize that with every step you take there is a moment when you are balancing on one leg. You are actually practicing a balancing exercise when you walk because you have to stand on one leg to swing the other one through. If it is a challenge to stand on two legs with your legs close together, how much of a challenge is it going to be to stand on one leg? Standing with your legs close together will help strengthen your inner thighs for better balance while you're walking.

If you like to lock your knees when you're standing upright, soften your knees just a little bit to feel more work with the hamstring muscles along the back of the thighs.

Now move up to your abdominals… If they are hanging out, you've got zero support for your lower back, and there's a good chance if you don't have back pain yet, it's going to affect you at some point. Your lower abs need to stay lifted, up, in, and back to help support the "front" of the spine, and work to lift your pelvis and torso up off the legs for a freer leg swing.

Ideally when we're in a vertical position there are three distinct curves of the spine: a slight arch in the neck, a C-Curve through the upper back, and another slight arch in the low back. If these 3 curves are in balance it is easier to move the spine in all directions, and we've got the shock absorption needed to support the back to walk and run.

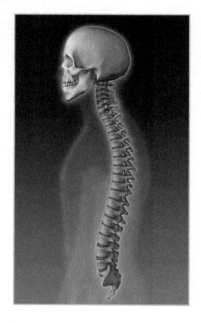

Sadly, poor posture habits and muscle imbalances due to lifestyle, sports, injuries, or lack of use contribute to pulling the body out of alignment. Retraining our muscles to work well is a part of what we're working on here with standing posture. Then the goal is to reinforce these new healthy movement habits while we practice our Pilates-Walk™ workouts.

Arms and Shoulders should ideally be hanging and relaxed by your sides. If you're one that likes to hike your shoulders up around your ears, or the stress of your day has them creeping upward, just thinking about just relaxing your shoulders may not be enough to make a difference. You may have to consciously engage the lower trapezius muscles to actively pull your shoulder blades down.

When your arms and shoulders go down, it cues your upper back, neck and head to shoot up! And voila – you'll be standing taller with better posture!

For more details, and tips on improving your posture, check out **Posture Principles for Health** at www.Centerworks.com.

Chapter 5

Breathing

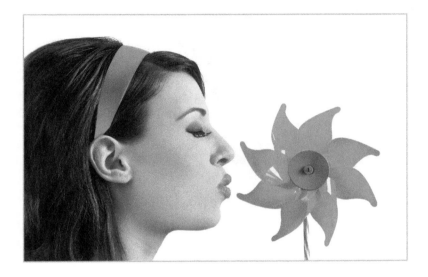

Breathing is the first thing we do in life and it will be the last. While it's great that we don't have to think about every breath we take to stay alive, paying attention to your breathing habits and working on improving them, can dramatically improve the amount of oxygen you will be able to take into your lungs to help nourish your brain and body.

There is a specific technique for Pilates breathing, it's called Posterio-Lateral breathing. This means breathing in so that the back of your rib cage fills with air. If you think about it, it makes sense to learn how to breathe into the back. Our lungs are located underneath the rib cage, and the rib cage spans the almost the whole torso.

If you just breathe into the front of your chest – you'll only be able to take small, shallow breaths – and chest breathing pulls your upper back out of alignment. If you practice abdominal breathing, your abs will pouch out on every inhale, which means with every breath you take you are losing the lower-abdominal support needed to help protect your lower back.

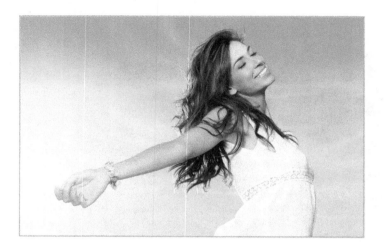

Good Pilates posterior-lateral breathing actually lengthens the natural curves of your spine on every inhale. Then, the goal is to strive to sustain some of that length on every exhale. When you breathe in, think about filling up your lungs from the bottom of your ribs all the way to the top of your spine, similar to filling a balloon with water.

If you tied a balloon to a sink and turned the water on, which end of the balloon fills up first, the bottom or the top? The bottom, right? This is exactly the same way you need to practice filling your lungs with air.

Your goal is to get comfortable filling your lungs with air from the bottom to the top, and the notice how this helps lift your rib cage UP off your hips to lengthen your spine. If this is done correctly, you will get taller and maintain the natural curves of your spine while practicing your Pilates posterior-lateral breathing.

PILATES *Walk*
PRACTICE EXERCISE
POSTERIO-LATERAL BREATHING

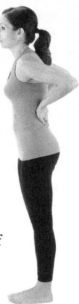

Because most of us are used to mainly breathing up into the chest or down into the belly – and we know that neither of these methods supports the back for good posture and a healthy spine – taking some time to focus on better breathing habits is critically important.

Remember: breathing into the back of the ribs from the bottom to the top will help improve your posture and give your back more support. Your goal is to practice the posterior-lateral Pilates style back breathing and get confident that with every breath you take you are filling up your lungs from the bottom to the top, lifting the ribs up off the hips, and improving your tall posture.

Posterio-Lateral Breathing

1. While standing tall with good posture; feet close together, knees soft, inner thighs working, shoulders relaxed, and ears over shoulders we are now going to practice breathing.

2. With every breath, inhale through your nose and exhale through your mouth. Feel the air come into the back of your rib cage.

3. If needed, place your fingers around the back of your ribs.

4. As you inhale, see if you can feel your ribs pull back in to your fingers, then exhale and feel your low abdominals pull up and in towards your back ribs.

The ribs lifting up and apart should cause your whole spine to lift up a little bit taller. Can you feel it?

It might be a challenge at first. This is brain and body work, so, right now, if your brain understands where to put the air, that's great. Know that it may take some practice to get your body to do it correctly and accept this new breathing habit as THE way to breathe.

Start with 10 deep breaths, or as many as you can without getting too dizzy. It's normal that deep breathing exercises can make you light-headed, but don't worry with time and practice the dizziness will go away. That will be a sign that your breathing habits are getting better.

One of my favorite ways to practice Pilates Posterio-Lateral breathing is with a winter scarf.

Bonus Exercise – Scarf Breathing

1. Take a winter scarf and place it around your back, holding onto it in the front with both hands.

2. As you inhale with the scarf around your ribs, feel your rib cage push back against the scarf as your lungs fill up with air, and your spine lifts taller.

3. As you exhale, lift your low abs up in and back towards the bottom edge of the scarf.

4. Repeat for 10 to 20 breaths.

Chapter 6

Low Bolts

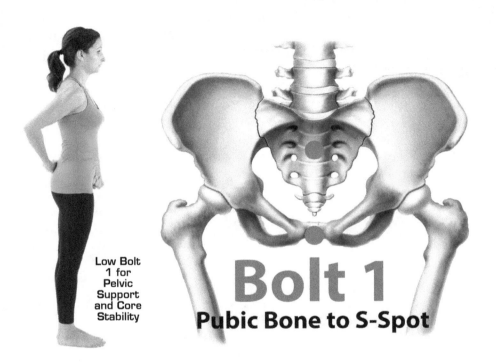

Low Bolt 1 for Pelvic Support and Core Stability

Bolt 1
Pubic Bone to S-Spot

Let's find and feel the benefits of low bolting. Imagine that you have two bolts at the bottom of your torso that give you support.

The first bolt is from the front of your pubic bone connecting up to the back of your pelvis. There is a little triangular bone, called the sacrum, at the bottom of your lower back. The goal is to think about bolting the front of your pubic bone to the back of your sacrum. Think about shortening and tightening this bolt a little bit; like you are screwing these two bones together. Don't worry about doing anything yet, we'll be practicing a bolting exercise in a moment. Right now, it's important that you have reference points to help connect the dots for successful bolting.

The second bolt is from two inches below your belly button up to the back of your rib cage. There are actually TWO second bolts, one on each side of the waist. The activation of Bolt #2 support lifts your lower abdominal muscles, up, in and back. Our low abdominal muscles tend to be lazy. If you happen to have lower back problems there's a good chance these muscles are weak. If the front of your belly is "hanging out," your pelvis tips forward and back goes into a big ol' banana sway!

Bolt 2 Two Inches Below the Navel to the Bottom Back Ribs

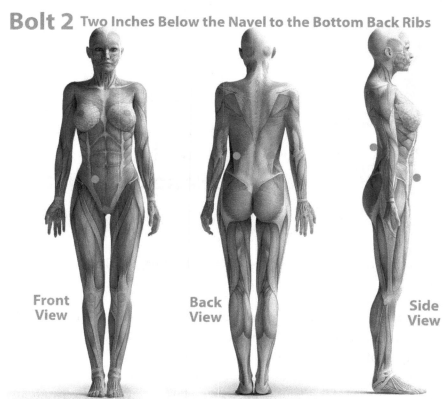

Front View

Back View

Side View

Bolt 2: Supports the low back, and defines the distance between the ribs and the hips

By finding and pulling that second bolt up, in and back from two inches below your belly button all the way up to the bottom of the back ribs, you'll notice that this helps lift and support the front of your body against the lower back.

Ideally, you should be using these two bolts all day long. Not just when you walk, not just when you sit, but all the time.

Bolt #2 is transverse abdominal muscle support. It helps keep our organs, intestines and everything held inside our body where they belong. Plus, bolt #2 is the abdominal muscle support for the front of the back, which is critical for a healthy spine.

PILATES *Walk*
PRACTICE EXERCISE
LOW BOLTS

Finding Bolt #1 – Seated

1. Sit in a chair with good posture, think about the front of your pubic bone pulling up and back on a diagonal to the back of your sacrum. When you find it, you may notice that it lifts you up just a tiny bit off your chair. It is not a big movement.

2. Bring these two bones a little closer together.

3. Feel the deep low support of bolt #1 – hold for 10-30 seconds then release.

4. Repeat 5 times.

5. There's a difference between doing it with your legs and really just doing it with the muscles in the pelvis.

6. The pubic bone to the sacrum is Bolt #1. If I say, "Bolt one," I'm looking for that really low support at the bottom of your pelvis. (*Above your pelvic floor and below your abs*)

Finding Bolt #2 – Seated

1. Still sitting in your chair with good posture and Bolt #1 engaged.

2. Find two inches below your belly button and pull it up, in, and back. Try to lift and press the lower abdominals up, in and back to the bottom of your back ribs, feeling the whole front of your abdomen flatten. And then relax it.

3. Engage bolt #2, hold for 10-30 seconds, then release.

4. Repeat 5 times.

Again, find Bolt #1, the pubic bone to the sacrum, and then bolt #2, two inches below the belly button to the back of the rib cage. You should notice that these contractions lift your body up a little bit off your chair, without gripping in the front of your hips.

Standing and Using Bolts 1 & 2

1. Now, stand up and try it. When you are walking, you need to have both bolts on.

2. Stand with your legs as close together as you are comfortable, a little soft at the knees.

3. Find Bolt #1, from the front of your pubic bone to the back of your sacrum and bring that up and in. Done correctly, it will "lift" your pelvis up off the legs.

4. Then Bolt #2, from two inches below your belly button on each side up to the back of your rib cage. To lengthen the wait and start lifting the ribs off the hips.

5. Pull these muscles up and in. Hold for 10-30 seconds and then release.

6. Repeat 5 times.

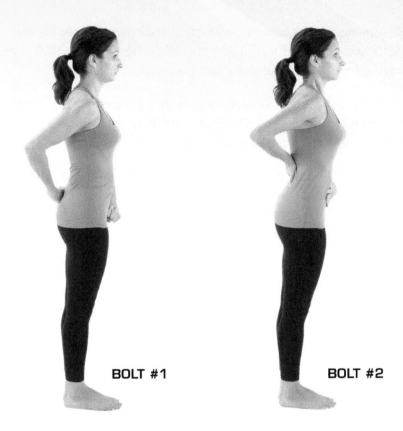

BOLT #1   BOLT #2

Ideally, you should be able to hold your bolts and breathe! Remember, the stomach muscles in the front are not actually connected to your lungs, they are completely separate! You should be able to keep your bolts on in the front and hold the support while breathing into the back of the rib cage.

Inhale and keep the bolts lifted while breathing into the back, exhale and see if you can squeeze a little more support out of Bolt #2. It is a lot of work, but we need this support! Not only to walk well, but for everything we do in life.

If you're finding it a challenge to simply sit or stand still, find your bolts for support and breathe. Can you imagine how much harder it's going to be to keep all this working AND walk? If you're feeling a little overwhelmed, hang in there.

The only way to get better is to practice, and you now have the rest of your life to fine-tune your technique. Just do the best you can today, and with time and practice, I promise it will get easier.

You can practice these small (*but powerful*) movements to find your bolts and breathe during any, or all, of your daily activities: Sitting at work, driving in the car, lying in bed, watching TV, exercising, etc.

I think you'll be surprised to find how quickly your body will embrace using this support, and when it is all working well, you'll discover how much easier it will be to maintain better body support when you walk.

Using the "S" Spot

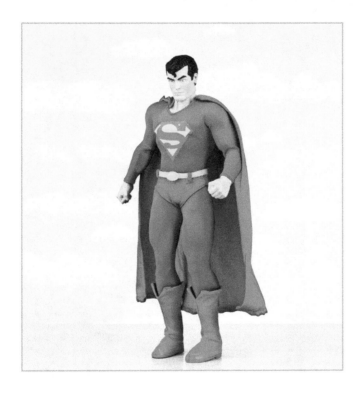

Consider the "S" spot as your "Super Support Spot." In Chapter 6 we talked about the sacrum, that little triangular-shaped bone at the bottom of your spine. It sits between your low back and your tailbone.

The sacrum actually looks a lot like the Superman logo, and your "S" spot is smack dab in the middle of your sacrum. Now that you know where your "S" spot is, use it as a reference point for your Bolt #1 support. Think about bolt #1 as a diagonal line from your pubic bone in the front, to your "S" spot in the back.

The "S" spot acts like a magnet connecting your back to your front. It is also your "S" spot in the back that propels you forward. Whether you are walking slowly or quickly, your "S" spot should be the driving force to move you forward.

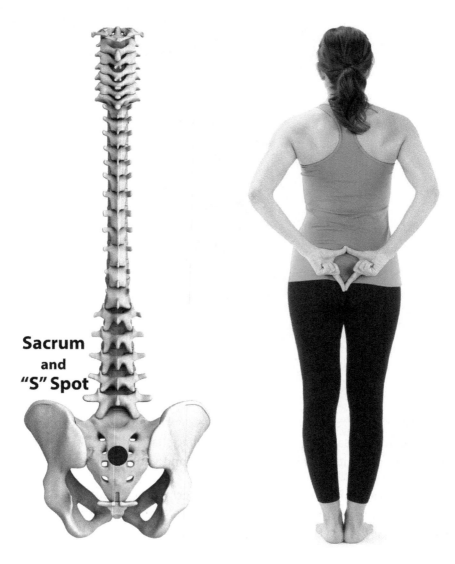

Sacrum
and
"S" Spot

PILATES *Walk*
PRACTICE EXERCISE
FINDING YOUR "S" SPOT

To find and activate your "S" Spot Seated

1. Sit up tall, find Bolt #1 and Bolt #2.

2. Now, see if you can find the magnet of the "S" spot. Did you feel a bit of "coming together" from the back to the front of the pelvis? It's almost like the sacrum moves forward a very tiny bit in between your hip bones.

3. Once you've got it, hold for 10-30 seconds, and relax.

4. Repeat 5 times.

You may not be able to feel it yet, but keep thinking about it periodically throughout your day because if your brain asks, "Hmm, where is this, can I find it?" and your brain keeps sending the message, sooner or later your body will figure it out and you'll be able to feel your S-spot activate.

To find the "S" Spot Standing

1. Stand up tall with good posture.

2. Find Bolt #1 (pubic bone to back of the sacrum), add Bolt #2 (two inches below your belly button to the back ribs).

3. Now see if you can find the little magnet of the "S" spot pressing forward just a little bit without losing the belly.

4. Hold for 10-30 seconds, and relax.

5. Repeat 5 times.

Can you find your "S" spot?

If you have trouble finding your it, place one hand in the middle of your lower back and place the other hand in the front on your low belly. With your core muscles, not your arms, bring your two hands closer together.

Your "S" spot is pulling the back hand to the front hand. It's a very small movement. When you keep the support in the front and you pull the back hand to the front hand THAT is the drive forward your "S" spot provides while you're walking.

Ok, let's take a look at how valuable your "S" Spot is for walking... Normally when people talk about walking technique they cue you to lead with your belly button.

I really don't want you to think about leading with your belly button because chances are you're going to stick out your abs so they can literally lead the way! If your belly is pooching out you will have zero back support, and limited mobility for your legs, hips, and spine for good gait.

But, when you keep your bolts on and lead with your "S" spot propelling you forward, you'll actually be pushing the body forward from the back, and maintaining good support in the front.

Good bolting and S-spot support will also allow a freer leg swing for better hip mechanics. When you walk with your "S" spot leading, you may even notice that your pace picks up a little bit. There's a chance that you'll walk a little faster because you have better support in your pelvis with your "S" spot engaged.

All of these little details can make a big difference for a healthy stride.

Chapter 8

Sexy Hips

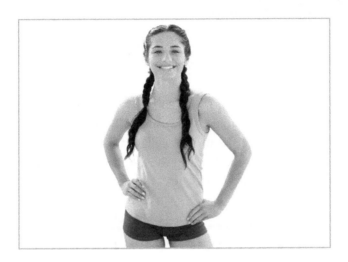

Move Your Sexy Hips! Whether you are male or female, we ALL need to move our hips when we walk. Women might swing them a little more than men, but men, I think your hips should be moving more when you walk, too, it's just better body mechanics.

Think about being a Diva on the runway. Okay men, maybe that's not the best image for you… But everyone should have some swinging going on with your hips when you walk.

This swinging action will help your lower back feel better and get stronger. The movement can be small but the hips need to be moving. Because if you hold your back stiff and keep your hips still when you walk, your lower back muscles will tighten, creating tension and, eventually, strain and pain in your SI joints and lower back.

When you walk and move your hips, it helps mobilize your lower back muscles so they get to work and release with every step. With a good sexy hip swing you are actually strengthening and relaxing the back muscles with every step you take.

Now the question is, which muscles are you using to get that sexy hip swing moving? It's not a wild, loose swing, but is done with control and support to allow free movement of the hips, back, and legs. What you are doing with your core is critical for a great sexy hip swing. I like the image of making the low front abdominals smile. We can put a smile on our face, so why not start smiling with our low abs?

Just thinking about it, can you start to feel your low abdominal muscles smiling? Can you actively make them smile? If you have to put smile on your face to get your low abs to lift, well, that's even better. And here's a hint – we've already covered finding these muscles, they are what you're using to find Bolt #2 (*But, for sexy hips, they lift one side at a time*)!

PILATES *Walk*
PRACTICE EXERCISE
FINDING YOUR SEXY HIP SWING

Finding Your Low Smile

1. Place your hands low on your belly and bring them up and out towards the front of your hip bones. It should feel like putting your hands in the pockets of your jeans, then sliding them up and out.

2. This is what you should be feeling as you your low abs smile. It will be VERY similar to finding Bolt #2, if both sides of your smile lift simultaneously.

3. Now, to get your sexy hips moving, you have to practice an alternate smile. One side of your smile comes up, and then the other side of your smile lifts. To get started, it might be easiest to start seated in a chair.

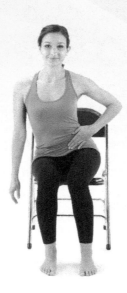

Seated Sexy Hip Exercise

1. Sit in a chair with your feet flat on the floor (about hip-width apart), and practice lifting your low smile.

2. Now, to introduce alternate smile, smile up one side of your belly. (*2 inches below your belly button on the right side lifts up towards the right back ribs*).

3. As you do this, the right butt cheek will come up off your chair a little bit. And then set it back down.

4. Do the other side: lift Bolt #2 (*2 inches below the belly button on the left side – up, in and back towards the left bottom ribs*). The left butt check will lift up off the chair.

5. The movement of the hips is like a teeter-totter from one sitting bone to the other.

6. Picking your feet up a little bit is cheating. Leave your feet down and feel your low abdominals lift to shift you weight from one tush to the other.

7. Keep your body tall and centered while your alternate low smile moves your sexy hips up and down.

8. Alternate sides for 5-10 repetitions.

Standing Sexy Hip Exercise

1. Are you ready to practice this Sexy Hip Swing, hip un-leveling exercise standing? Let's stand on your feet and give it a try. To practice this movement standing still, you'll have to bend one knee to achieve the sexy hip movement.

2. Stand with both legs close together in your good, tall posture position.

3. As the right low abs smile, the left knee bends. This should shorten the distance between the right hip and ribs and lengthen the waist on the left side.

4. Straighten the left knee to return the hips to a level, even position.

5. Now lift the left low abs up while bending the right knee, alternating the action – left hip and ribs get closer together, right side of the waist gets a stretch.

6. Be sure as you bend each knee that both feet stay flat on the floor.

7. Maintain abdominal support throughout the exercise, and always come back to two straight legs so that your pelvis is level and even before alternating sides.

8. This is a side-to-side motion. Be sure you're not "twerking" your butt cheek to one back corner behind you as you un-level your hips.

9. Alternate sides 5-10 times.

Remember the "S" spot in the middle of the sacrum? That "S" spot is the pivot point for your Sexy Hip Swing. Visualize a little dot on your "S"-spot. Your goal is to move your alternate smile around this spot. Try not to let your "S" spot swing side to side with your hips. Strive to keep your "S" spot still and make your pelvis swing around it. You

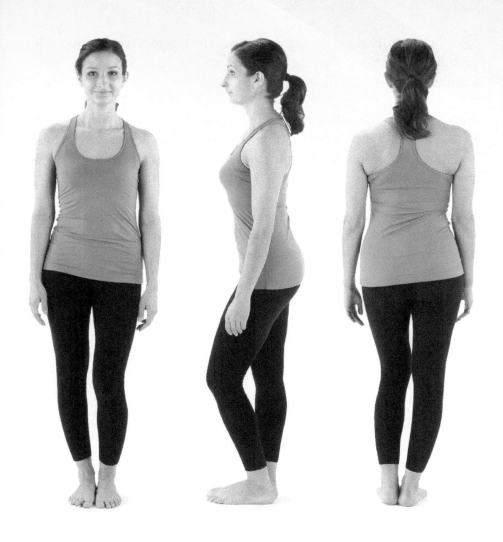

might notice that to accomplish this task, it will require a little more muscle work from your low abs to support the movement.

As you practice this one-knee bend, hip un-leveling exercise to warm up your sexy hip swing, be sure that both feet stay flat on the floor. As one knee bends it shortens the leg and causes the hip to lower on that side and lift on the other, pivoting the pelvis around your "S" spot and your standing leg.

Ideally, you want feel this very same hip movement when you walk. Of course there is a little more movement involved than just un-leveling for your sexy hip swing, but learning how to get this movement first will make everything else easier.

What's really great about this preparatory sexy hip swing exercise is that it allows you to practice the feeling of swinging your hips without worrying about everything else that needs to be moving.

Chapter 9

Leg Swing

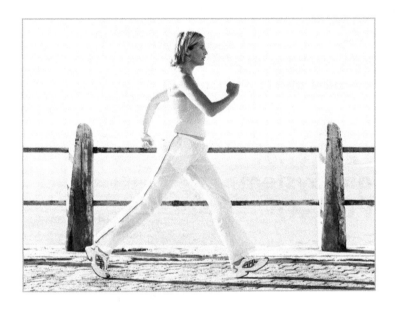

If it wasn't complicated enough, we are now going to talk about parts of the body we can't see, but are still crucial to walking well.

It's critical that you learn to use the muscles on the BACK of your body to move you forward. This is achieved by activating your Posterior Oblique System (POS). The Posterior Oblique System is the muscle support system, or firing pattern, through the back of your body. It makes up half of what is needed to balance the body from the front to the back, and provides the power to propel you forward to walk and run.

Since we can't see what is behind us, we don't think too much about what is going on back there. But, we can't just forget about it because the biggest muscles we've got are behind us!

Your Posterior Oblique System forms an X-pattern of support along the back of the body. The POS firing pattern is:

1. Hamstrings
2. Glutes
3. Opposite side Low Back
4. Same side Latissimus Dorsi (or Lat)

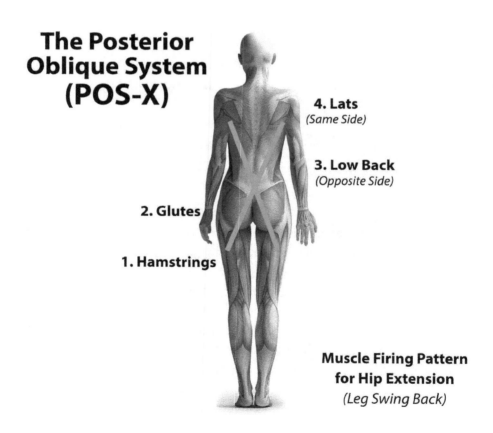

The Posterior Oblique System (POS-X)

4. Lats
(Same Side)

3. Low Back
(Opposite Side)

2. Glutes

1. Hamstrings

Muscle Firing Pattern for Hip Extension
(Leg Swing Back)

The right Hamstrings, right Glute, left side Low Back, left side Lat make up one side of the X, and the left Hamstring, left Glute, right side Low Back, and right Lat make up the other side of the X.

In my experience working with bodies in the health and fitness field for more than 30 years, I have noticed that the average person on the street today tends to walk with the legs more in front of the body than behind them. This makes it much more difficult to find and use the pattern of the Posterior Oblique System (POS) support for a healthy stride. We have to learn how to get the legs to swing farther behind us!

Having a stride where the leg swings more in front of the body with every step means tight hip flexors, over-developed quads, weak hamstrings, an increased risk of Sacro-illiac (SI joint) problems, and low back pain. In part, our lifestyle habits are to blame for this muscle imbalance because we are either sitting in a chair at our computers all day with our hips flexed. And/or, we make poor shoe choices (*flip-flops, clogs, and strapless sandals*) that shorten our stride and unknowingly cause us to walk without taking our legs completely behind us.

When we stand up and start to walk, our legs tend to stay in front of the body because that's what we are used to doing. In addition, poor shoe choices have us taking short little steps because our shoes might fall off. Finally, as we get older, because we haven't really been using our POS, lack of hip strength and balance become an issue, causing us to take smaller and wider steps to avoid falling. This combination of bad movement habits (*that you probably don't even realize are happening*) are setting you up for a stride that lacks support from your POS. Smaller, shorter steps increase the gap for muscle imbalances, and increase the risk of injury or chronic pain. A longer stride can help keep your muscles stronger, your POS active, and your body in better balance. It becomes a matter of increasing awareness about our daily habits, and finding ways to actively strengthen your Posterior Oblique System.

Walking happens to be one of the most effective and efficient forms of exercise for training your POS, but only if you are walking with good technique! Poor posture and bad movement habits are only going to reinforce what you've been doing wrong. Your Pilates-Walk™ training is going to help you find and feel the right muscles working to get that X-pattern of your POS system fired up and working well to support you for walking and everything else you do in life.

Using the Posterior Oblique System (POS) When You Walk

When you step forward to walk, it is important that you have a long enough stride to be able to engage your Posterior Oblique System and feel the muscles in the back of your body working. The POS chain goes from the hamstring muscles along the back of the thigh, through to the Glutes (*back of your butt*), across your body to the lower back on the opposite side, and then up to the shoulder blade and the back of the arm. It truly is a giant X of support on a diagonal line through the back of your body.

If you do not take a big enough step, you cannot get these POS muscles in the back of your body to do their job. First, you need to have a stride that is long enough to activate these muscles. And secondly, you've got to have your leg, hip, pelvis, low back, shoulder, and arm working together correctly for proper body mechanics to get the work to cross over from the right to left, or left to right, to access your X.

PILATES *Walk*
PRACTICE EXERCISE
TO ACCESS THE POS AND
IMPROVE LEG SWING

Until you are confident with balance, do this exercise holding on to a chair, railing, or counter-top for balance.

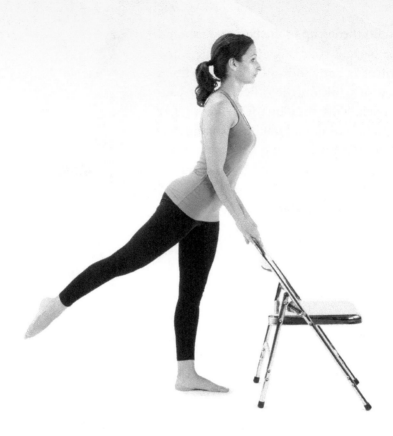

Standing One Leg Lift to the Back

1. Stand on one leg and point the toes of the other leg down to the back behind you.

2. Then, squeeze with the back of the thigh and lift the whole leg up off the floor a little bit, and lower it back down.

3. Again, squeeze with the back of your leg and lift it up just a little bit, and lower it back down.

4. Lift and lower your leg to the back 5-10 times.

5. Switch and do the same exercise on the other leg.

As you lift the leg up to the back, you should feel the back of your thigh (*hamstrings*), the back of your butt, and – if all goes well – a little bit of work on the other side of your lower back. This shouldn't feel like a lot of work, and there should not be any pain. Your goal is to use this Standing Leg Lift to the Back exercise to wake up the connection for the correct firing pattern for your Posterior Oblique System.

For now, it's important to keep your hips and shoulders facing straight ahead. If you lift your leg up to the back and your same side hip hikes up, you are going to feel the work it on the same side of your back, which is incorrect. If both hips stay forward, you will find it easier to get to the crossover position for the X-pattern of muscle for firing your Posterior Oblique System to activate correctly.

As the leg is lifting, think about lifting the whole leg, not just the heel and the lower leg. If you just lift the heel it is a different exercise than if you lift the whole leg. The movement to lift the leg is the ball of the thigh bone moving in the socket of the pelvis. If you lead from the foot to lift, you'll be bending the knee and initiating the lift from the wrong end of the leg. Can you feel a difference? It's that whole-leg strength that you want to work on to activate your POS.

Please note that just by standing here, using the chair for balance and practicing this Leg Lift to the Back exercise, you are working on a longer stride. Having the strength and freedom of movement to swing the leg farther behind you, means that you are working on being able to take a bigger step forward (*and the result will be that the other leg is farther back*). Plus, when you walk, the leg lifts off the floor behind you before you bend the knee and swing the leg through, just like this one leg lift to the back exercise.

Prone One Leg Lift Back Exercise

Getting started, you can also do this Leg Lift to the Back exercise lying on your stomach. This can make it easier to feel if you are twisting your hips and/or using the same side low back instead of the opposite side. In this position, you can feel if your "S" spot and both hip bones stay on the floor in front of you while the leg lifts to the back.

Prone One Leg Lift Back Exercise

1. Lay on your stomach, legs together, arms by your sides, tip of your nose on the mat.

2. Lengthen your tailbone to your heels and lift your low abs for support.

3. Pull your shoulders down to lengthen your upper spine and float your head up off the mat.

4. Inhale to lift your left leg and right arm activating the POS.

5. Exhale to lower the arm and leg, alternate sides.

6. Repeat 5 to 10 times.

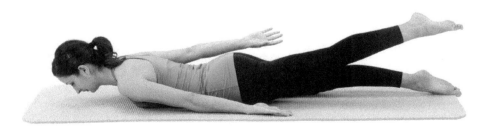

Is it a challenge to find your POS in a standing position? Does lying down on your stomach to practice the Prone One Leg Lift Exercise bother your back? Don't worry, you're not alone...It's important that you find exercise that can safely help you develop this strength.

There are some very effective ways to work on Posterior Oblique action and hip strength with the Pilates Arc Barrel. If you are interested in learning more ways to work on hip and shoulder mechanics, I highly recommend you get a Pilates Arc Barrel, it's a great tool for at-home training. You'll find lots of easy-to-learn hip strengthening exercises in my book, *"A Barrel of Fun,"* available at Centerworks.com.

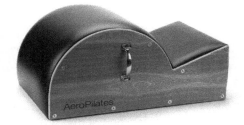

Chapter 10

Feet

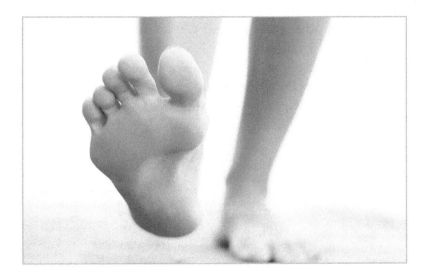

Feet are so very, very important. We tend to think that feet are just down there and, because we're standing, walking or running, that they're doing their job. But that's not always the case. Our muscles do what we've trained them to do. Our patterns and habits dictate which muscles we use and how well we use them. Paying attention to your feet and ankles can make a HUGE difference in walking well and staying injury-free! If you want better balance, body control, and improved posture, you'd be well advised to start paying more attention to your feet.

Your feet and ankles are what push you forward. If you take a little tiny step, your ankles and feet do not work very hard; they almost stay locked in the same position. If you take a longer step, the whole foot and ankle has to move. With every step forward you should be going from a flexed foot, thru a flat foot, to pointed toes. That flex-to-the-point action rolls through the whole foot, and the final push-off that propels you forward is with the muscle under the ball of the feet and the big toe.

Our arches need to be both supple and rigid to provide the lever action to roll through the foot. If you have flat feet, you have weak arches: if you have high arches, chances are some parts of your arch may be overworking, and other parts of your feet are underdeveloped. If your ankles roll inward or outward, there is a muscle imbalance not only in your feet, but also in your ankles, and calves. If you have plantar fasciitis, bunions, hammer toes, or any of the other foot issues mentioned above, or if you are prone to ankle sprains and strains, there is a lot you can do to improve your foot fitness which in turn will help you walk with a healthier stride.

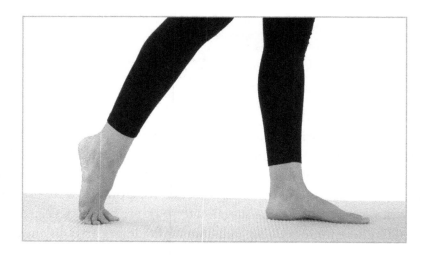

Here are two simple foot fitness exercises to help you focus on the alignment and muscle action of your feet and ankles. This first exercise is from my book *Fantastic Feet! Exercises to Strengthen the Ankles, Arches, and Toes.*

PILATES *Walk*
PRACTICE EXERCISE
FOOT FITNESS

Seated Flex and Point Exercise

1. Sit with your feet out in front of you. Legs together, knees and toes pointing straight up.

2. Flex your feet and reach the heels away from you. This "flexed" ankle position is the foot position for the "heel-strike" of the forward foot in your stride.

3. Next, point the ankles as far as you can move them away from you, then point the toes.

4. Release the toes and flex at the ankle, reaching the heels away.

5. Continue to alternate between flexing and pointing the ankle, arches, and toes 5-10 times.

Easy Version – both feet point and flex at the same time.
Challenge – Right points while the left flexes – alternate feet (*the flipper-foot action of gait*).

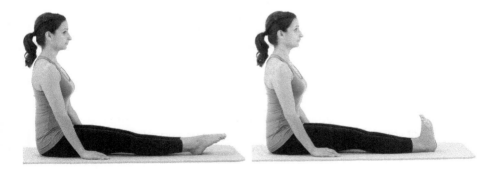

If you get a stretch in the back of your calf when you flex, it's a bonus. This is a good exercise to practice without shoes on because you want to practice using your whole foot (*ankle, arches, and toes to do the movement*). After you point the ankle, the toes flipper over the edge to point too. As you flipper the toes down, you should feel the muscles along the sole of your foot working. It's pretty normal to feel your feet cramp on this exercise. If your arches or toes cramp quickly, the muscles may be weak. Practicing this exercise will help them get stronger and eventually, the foot cramps will go away.

This seated flex and point exercise is a great place to practice what your ankles should be doing when you walk without having to worry about your balance. It also allows you the opportunity to watch your feet to be sure everything is staying in good alignment while you're moving the ankles, arches, and toes.

Standing Calf Stretch to Flipper Toes Exercise

1. Stand in a good, tall, upright position. You may want to hold on to the back of a chair or wall for balance.

2. Take the right leg back about a stride's length behind you and bend the front knee. The back leg should be straight with the heel pressing down into the floor to start (lunge position).

3. All of your toes should be facing straight ahead (not off to the side). You do not have to be on a tightrope; take your legs hip-width apart to help with balance.

4. Rise up onto the ball of your back foot. Go all the way up onto your tippy-toes and flipper the toes over to a strong pointed position. Then, roll back down through the foot (from the ball to the heel), pressing the back heel into the floor.

5. The front knee stays bent for balance.

6. Keep your belly up for good support.

7. Your "S" spot should be moving forward as you rise onto the ball of your back foot, flipper the toes to point, and roll back down to press the heel into the floor for a calf stretch.

8. If you have a hard time balancing, take your feet apart just a little bit wider.

9. Rise up and practice your flipper toes, to calf stretch 5-10 times and then switch legs.

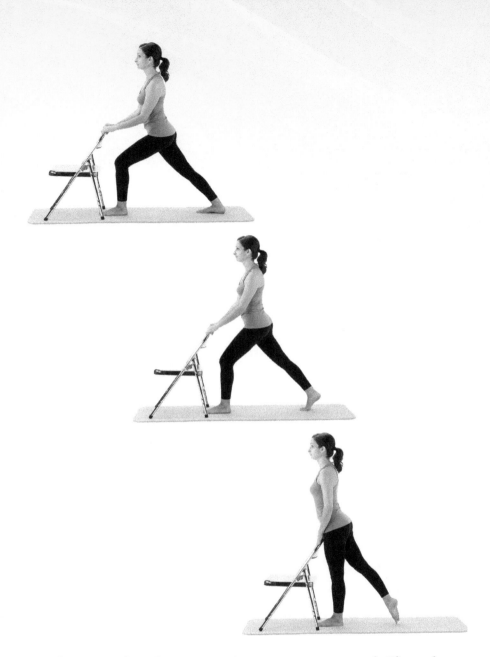

Use these two foot fitness exercises to get you started. If you know your feet need more training time to stay healthy, I'd encourage you to check out the Foot Fitness section at Centerworks.com for more helpful Foot-Care resources.

Chapter 11

Core Support

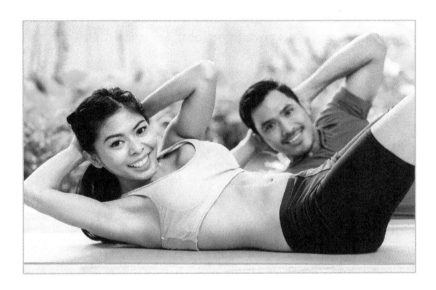

Have you ever put this much thought into how all the parts and pieces of your body are designed to work together? Or really considered what healthy movement habits your body needs for optimal biomechanics to walk with ease?

I'm guessing you probably were just like me before I started discovering the benefits of Pilates. I thought I knew my body, and could make it do anything I wanted...until I had a mentor that pointed out all my weaknesses and muscle imbalances! Most of my clients feel the same way in the Pilates studio when they start re-learning how to walk with Pilates-Walk movement principles: it's like they've never walked a day in their life! But changes can happen quickly once you better understand what you're working on and why.

There is A LOT to pay attention to when you're walking (*like everything from your head to your toes!*), and just like doing Pilates, walking really needs to have proper support from your core. What are your abs doing when you walk? Are they hanging out and leading the way or lifting up, in, and back to support your lower back and torso? Do you realize how important core strength is to support both your arms and legs as they swing when you walk?

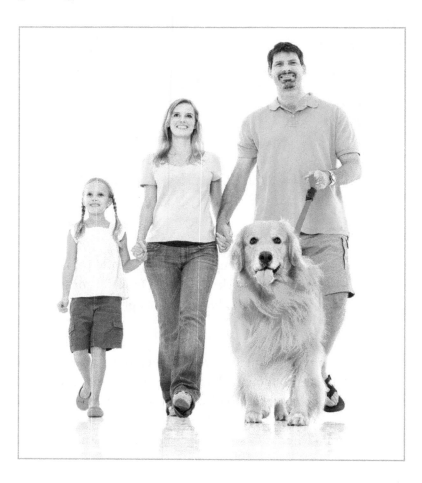

Abdominals are a hot topic for health improvement. Everybody knows they're important. Now the question is, how well are yours working?

So far we have covered exercises and concepts to find and use your two low bolts (*Bolt #1 – pubic bone to "S" spot, and Bolt #2 – 2 inches below the belly to the back of the ribs*) We've discussed the low ab smile, and alternate smile to help with your sexy hip swing and hip un-leveling, and the importance of finding and using your "S" spot to lead the way. ALL of this is working on improving your core support for standing, sitting, and walking!

Here is one more easy abdominal exercise you can add to your workouts to strengthen your abdominals and mobilize your spine. The Standing Roll Down the Wall exercise is great because gravity is helping you bend the spine forward. And, with your back against a wall, you've got something to pull your abs up, in, and back against to find even more support. Plus, you don't have to worry about balance when you're leaning against a wall.

Ab work is great lying on the floor too, and there are LOTS of Pilates Mat exercises that have you lying on your back with your head and shoulders curled up off the floor. However, sometimes lying on the floor isn't convenient, especially if you're heading out for a walk. And for a lot of people doing crunches and sit-ups only seem to lead to neck strain and back pain, not developing stronger abdominals. Good technique matters…

Once you know how to work and release the right muscles, you will get a lot more from your core for regular sit-ups and Pilates ab work. Meanwhile, this Standing Roll Down can be a great exercise to start with. If you think about it, standing against a wall, keeping everything pulling back to the wall, and rolling forward is like doing a sit-up from a standing position only you're using gravity to help you. It's not often when we exercise that gravity is our friend!

PILATES *Walk*
PRACTICE EXERCISE
IMPROVE CORE SUPPORT

Standing Roll Down Exercise on the Wall

Keep in mind, this exercise is not about working your abs so hard that they are cramping, burning, or too tired to really work well. It's about finding the support with your abdominals that you really should be using ALL DAY LONG! Especially when you're walking!

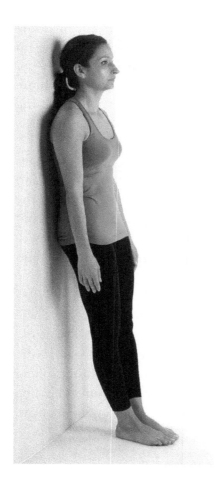
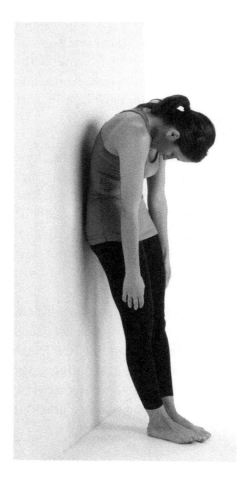

Standing Roll Down Exercise on the Wall

1. Stand with your back against a wall.

2. You can start with your legs hip-width apart, but over time, I encourage you to stand with your legs and feet close together.

3. Be sure your feet and knees are in a parallel position with everything facing straight ahead.

4. In your tall standing position, keep your whole back firmly pressed against the wall – it's best to start with your feet fairly far away from the wall to make it easier to keep your back ON the wall (*as your back gets more flexible, and your low abs get stronger, you will be able to progressively scoot your feet closer to the wall, until they are only 2-6 inches out*).

5. Inhale and lift your back up tall, exhale and nod the chin to the chest to begin bending forward and peeling the back away from the wall one segment at a time. The farther forward you bend, the more your abdominals need to pull up, in, and back to the wall.

6. To start you may only bend forward to the bottom of the shoulder blades. As you get comfortable keeping your support, continue bending forward to the waist.

7. Strive to keep your low bolts on, and your low back against the wall.

7. Continue breathing naturally as you bend forward.

9. Inhale and exhale to start with the low abdominals and sequentially roll up from the bottom to the top to return to your tall "back against the wall" standing position.

10. Keep your low abs pressed firmly to the wall as you stand up tall. Feel your arms and shoulders drop down and relax as your chest, neck and head lift up to finish tall.

11. Repeat this exercise 3-5 times.

If it's easy to maintain your abdominal support and sequentially roll down and back up, scoot your feet a little closer to the wall on each repetition to challenge yourself. If you need more to strengthen your core, get yourself into Pilates for cross-training. Both Pilates Matwork and Pilates equipment training can be valuable for helping you improve not only your core strength, but every part of your body that's needed to walk well!

One more core training exercise that definitely needs to be in your weekly workouts is the Criss-Cross from the Series of 5 in Pilates Matwork. If you know the exercise, do the full version. Otherwise, start with the modified version outlined below:

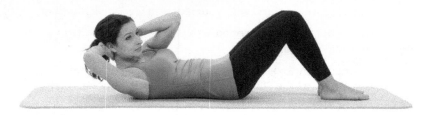

Criss-Cross Abs

1. Lay on your back, legs together, knees bent, feet flat on the floor.

2. Place your hands behind your head to help support the neck.

3. Take one full breath, inhale and exhale to curl the head and shoulders up off the mat *(ideally to the bottom tips of the shoulder blades)*.

4. Rotating from the waist up, twist the spine to the right and center, then left and center. Stay in the curled-up position as you pass through center. Strive to make the twist happen from the waist and only use the arms and shoulders to support the weight of the head.

5. If you're elbows are flapping, you're pulling with your arms to twist, not using your abs! You may move as slowly or quickly as you'd like, as long as you're maintaining a good position and moving with control.

6. lternate sides for 8-20 repetitions.

7. Breathe throughout the exercise. You have a couple of choices for breath patterns:

Beginner Breathing – Inhale twist, Exhale center, OR Exhale twist, Inhale Center. Ideally it should be easy for you to breathe both ways, so I'd encourage you to practice BOTH of these breathing patterns.

Intermediate/Advanced – Inhale twist right AND left, Exhale twist right AND left.

Note: It's very important that your hips and pelvis stay still. The rotation to twist is from the waist up to effectively strengthen your oblique abdominals and the muscles that rotate your spine.

Three Tips to Challenge Your Criss-Cross Exercise

1. Alternate one knee to elbow
2. Hold both legs up to table-top position
3. Bend one knee to the chest and extend the other leg away

If you're looking for a quick cross-training workout you can do in 10 minutes or less as a warm-up or cool-down for your Pilates-Walk workouts – check out the e-book ***Pulse Power™ The Daily Dozen 10 Minute Pulse-Power Workout Plan*** on Amazon or at centerworks.com. This fast and effective training program starts out with four excellent core strengthening exercises, and continues into a quick whole-body workout that can help reinforce what you're learning to find and use for your Pilates-Walk™ Workouts.

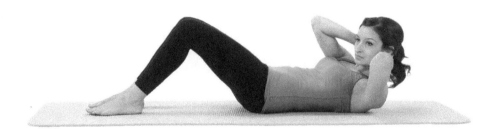

Chapter 12

Arms & Shoulders

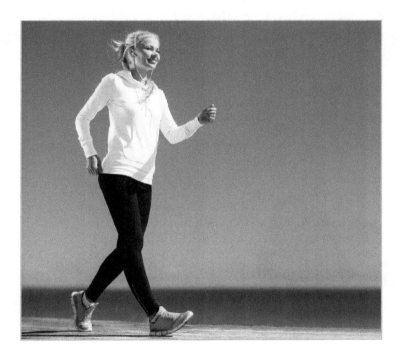

Just like your leg swing, the arms and shoulders need to SWING freely for a healthy stride. If one arm is going forward, the other arm should be going backward; in part, this is what helps counter-balance your upper body when you walk. Your arm swing also helps increase speed, assists with improving core strength, and plays a part in keeping your spine healthy. Whether you choose to swing with bent arms or straight arms, it's important to learn how to swing the whole arm from the shoulder.

If your shoulders are hiked up around your ears, aside from creating unnecessary tension in your neck and shoulders, it's inefficient for a healthy arm swing. If your shoulders are UP and stuck, you'll end up thinking you're swinging the arms, when in fact you're only moving your forearms and just swinging from the elbows. Your arm swing shouldn't be just the forearm; it's the whole arm.

Remember earlier, when I said that we are so used to focusing on what is in front of us that we typically don't pay attention to what's going on behind us? Since we don't have eyes in the back of our heads we can't see

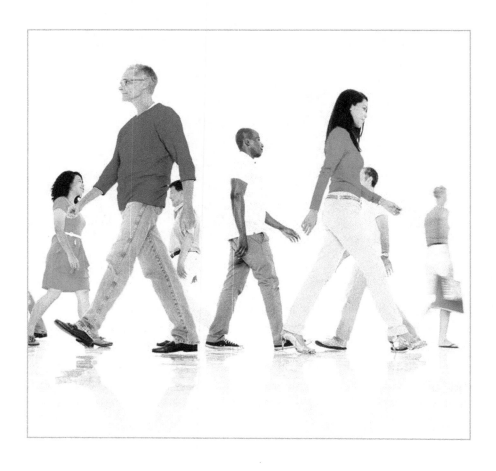

what we are doing when it's happening behind the body. We've got to improve our body awareness!

The concept of a healthy arm swing is similar to what we've already discussed for your leg swing. Chances are, if your leg swing is more in front of the body, your arm swing will be doing the same thing. This means the front of the arms and shoulders are getting stronger, and the back of the arms and shoulders are getting weaker, creating an imbalance that is widening the gap between your dominant and weaker muscles.

The arm swing to the back is what engages the endpoint for the posterior oblique system. You can practice your arm swing sitting or standing still to become more aware of swinging the whole arm from the shoulder, and making sure that the arms are swinging evenly forward and back.

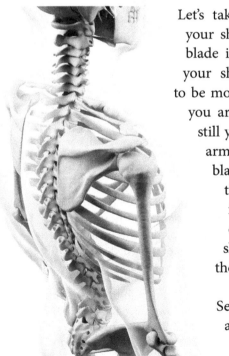

Let's take a quick moment to look at your shoulder anatomy. Your shoulder blade is attached to your arm. BOTH your shoulder blade AND arm need to be moving for a healthy arm swing. If you are holding your shoulder blades still you cannot effectively move your arms. Learn to let your shoulder blades move with your arms and the swing of the arms will be a lot freer. When the exercise is done correctly, you should feel your shoulder blades gliding around the rib cage as the arms swing.

Set your book down for a minute and practice your arm swing...

PILATES *Walk*
PRACTICE EXERCISE
ARMS AND SHOULDERS

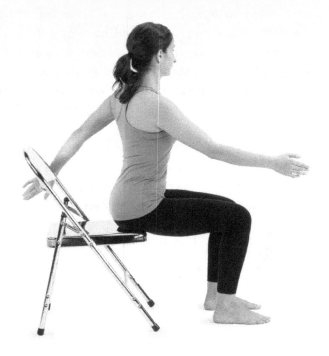

Seated Arm Swing

1. As you're sitting in your chair, (*or standing*) and swinging your arms can you feel the shoulder blades moving a little bit? There is a moment when both arms drop down by your sides, this helps drop all that unnecessary neck and shoulder tension out of your body.

2. Be careful that your arm swing is not too high to the front. It is better for the arm in the front to be lower and the arm in the back to be a little higher, but if possible, you're goal is an even arm swing with the front and back arms at the same height.

Do you have a bent-arm swing, or a straight-arm swing? Either is perfectly okay for walking!

A good rule of thumb with a bent-arm swing is for your thumb to be at chin- or nose-level in the front so you can get the back arm higher.

For a straight-arm swing the front arm should lift to about belly-button height. If the front arm stays lower and the back arm goes higher this will help increase the flexibility of your arms and shoulders, strengthen the back of the shoulder and upper arm, and help you develop a more well-balanced body.

As your arms are swinging strive to keep them in line with your shoulders. Some people walk with a crazy arm swing that goes side-to-side instead of front-to-back. Try not to let your arms cross your mid-line as they're swinging.

There is one more very important thing to pay attention to for a good arm swing.

What do you notice is happening to your spine while you're swinging your arms? Does your back stay stiff and torso square to the front? Or does your torso rotate? (*A rotating torso means you're twisting and rotating your spine*).

A big part of maintaining whole-body health is keeping your spine healthy. Ideally our back should bend forward, sideways, backwards and twist. Having the ability to move your spine freely in all ranges of motion helps keeps your body strong, fit, and flexible. When you do the sexy hip movement and the alternate low ab smile, you're actually helping the lower back feel better by strengthening the core and stretching the back with a side-bending lateral movement. As a part of the arm swing, there needs to be some rotational movement happening for the spine and rib cage. This twisting motion helps strengthen the oblique abdominals and releases any unnecessary tension held in the torso.

Standing Arm Swing

1. Stand with good tall posture and begin to swing your arms. Can you feel the shoulder blades move, the whole-arm swing, and notice a little bit of rotation of the spine?

2. As the right arm swings forward the right shoulder goes forward, which means the left shoulder and arm will swing back. It is not a huge amount of rotation, but you should feel the whole spine twist, from the waist up.

3. Focus on feeling the turn initiate from your belly button and be sure your criss-cross Ab muscles are working to help turn the torso.

4. Allow the whole rib cage to rotate with the arm swing.

5. Pay attention to feeling the whole arms swing an even distance to the front and back.

6. Take 30 seconds to 1 minute to just stand still and swing your arms freely like a pendulum.

Can you feel the shoulders drop? Are your arms at an even swinging height to the front and back and not crossing the mid-line? Can you feel the rotation of the spine and the rib cage?

Are you starting to feel a little more warmed up, just by swinging your arms, rotating your spine, and using your Obliques? Isn't it amazing how focusing on moving just your arms can get the blood pumping!

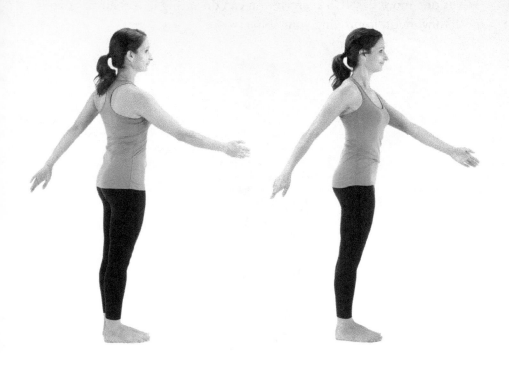

Practicing this Standing Arm Swing exercise can help improve your body awareness and make you really feel what the back arm is doing. Starting to notice that little bit of spine rotation and Oblique support through your torso is really important too. You can practice your arm swing anywhere! If you're feeling blah in the middle of the day, sit or stand up and take 30 seconds to swing your arms from the shoulders and twist your spine to enjoy a moment of movement to re-energize your body.

Here's one more BONUS exercise you can do sitting in a chair or at your desk to work on improving your spine twist.

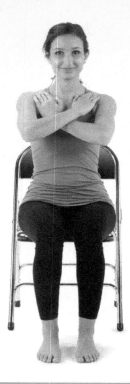

Seated Simple Twist Exercise

1. Sit up nice and tall on the front edge of your chair.

2. Plant your feet firmly on the floor, legs hip-width apart.

3. Take your arms and cross them across your chest to help keep your shoulder blades down and spread wide.

4. Start turning your torso from your belly button up as far around to one side as you are comfortable twisting. Then, pull your belly button back around to face center.

5. Practice this Seated Twist 5-10 times, alternating sides.

This twisting movement requires a little bit of your low smile on one side to initiate the turn, while the opposite side of the back pushes the other side of the spine forward.

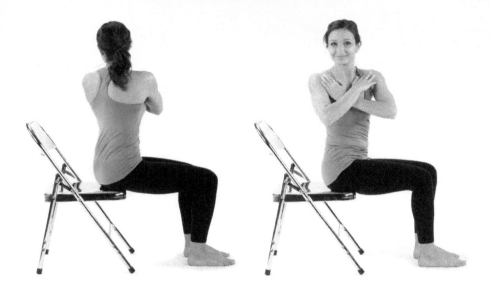

- To Twist LEFT – Left low abs, Right low back – middle back – upper back.
- To Twist RIGHT – Right low abs, Left low back – middle back – upper back.

Start with your low spine turning from the waist up, the middle spine rotates the bottom of the rib cage, the upper back and breastbone turn to take the shoulders farther around, and finally the head and neck turn.

Start back at the bottom of the spine to un-rotate and return to center.

You will not twist the spine as far around when you walk as you do with this exercise, but it's a great one to feel the front and the back of the body working together to achieve rotation. This same muscle action happens when you walk and swing your arms; the range of motion is just smaller and the movement is much faster.

Chapter 13

Putting It All Together

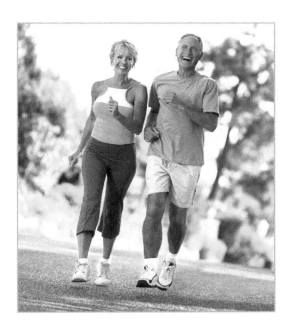

Let's take a quick review of everything we've covered and why it's important to pay attention to what every single piece of your body is doing with every step you take in order to develop healthy movement habits and get the best benefits possible from your walking workouts.

Review of Pilates-Walk™ Concepts

Good Posture – Think about standing tall, and maintaining the natural curves of the spine. When you are supported from the ground up, your body will be in better alignment, causing less wear and tear on your joints, and more joint space for free and easy movement.

Breathing – Practice Pilates-style posterio-lateral breathing techniques to fill up your lungs from the bottom to the top. Breathe in to your back and support your low belly while elongating the natural curves of the spine.

Bolt #1 – The pubic bone to the sacrum on a long, up-and-together diagonal. The muscle support here creates a sandwich of support for the pelvis and helps lift the pelvis up off the legs for a freer leg swing.

Bolt #2 – Two inches below the belly button to the back of your rib cage. Remember there are actually TWO Bolt #2's – one on each side of the navel. This support lengthens your waist, supports the low back, and defines the distance between your hips and ribs.

The "S" Spot – The "S" Spot is a little magnet of support in the middle of your sacrum. This is the spot that propels you forward (*from the back*) to walk, and it's the pivot point for your sexy hip swing.

Low Smile – Low Abs – Core work not only helps support your back, but frees up the back and hips for better body mechanics and gait. Your alternate low smile is what assists with the un-leveling of your hips for your sexy hip swing.

POS – The Posterior Oblique System is the X-Pattern of support through the BACK of the body. The muscle firing pattern is Hamstring, Glute, Opposite Side Low Back, Same Side Lat. (*Right Hamstring, Right Glute, Left Low Back, Left Lat.*) In order to effectively get your POS working, your stride length must be long enough to have one leg swing behind your body as you move forward. Strengthening your POS system will help reduce low back pain, alleviate SI joint problems, and help release grippy, tight hip flexors. As the leg swings forward, the hinge is where the leg meets the pelvis; as the leg swings back, the hinge is that side of the pelvis all the way to the top front of the hip bone AND the leg, with a stable "S" Spot.

Feet and Ankles – The calf stretch to flipper toes action is helping to mobilize the ankle joint and strengthen the arch of the foot. Having good foot and ankle alignment and getting your toes involved will improve your posture, balance, and body control. Also remember, your ankles, arches, and toes provide the back foot's final push off the ground to propel you forward for a healthy stride.

Arm Swing & Torso Rotation – A good arm swing involves the whole arm, not just the forearm! The shoulder blades swinging are a part of a healthy arm swing, too. Strive to swing the arms as far to the back as they go to the front, and let the swing of the arms help turn the torso to find and use the Oblique Abdominals. Ideally, the spine rotation comes from the waist up, and the shoulders and arms "ride along" with the twist, without the arms crossing past the mid-line.

Putting It All Together for an Effective Pilates-Walk Workout

Integrating all of these concepts is A LOT to think about and pay attention to with every step! Chances are you're not going to be able to incorporate all of these tweaks to your technique at once. Some movements may be fairly easy for your body to figure out, others might take some time and practice to get good at. To get started, on your next walk, pick ONE of the Pilates-Walk training concepts to pay attention to for 2-5 minutes and then switch to the next one, and the next…. By the end of a 30 minute Pilates-Walk workout you will have cycled through every part of your body that you need to focus on for a more efficient stride.

Or, you can take an entire walk and focus on one new healthy movement habit. Then, on your next walk, pick something else to add while maintaining the improvements from the previous workout. Keep adding elements. If something starts to slip, go back and work on that one concept again until it becomes a familiar habit.

Personally, I like rotating and practicing all of my concepts during one walking workout. Usually I'll decide that I'm going to focus on my S-Spot leading for one block, then I might go for the next three light poles feeling my low smile and sexy hips, then from the fire hydrant to the car on the corner paying attention to my POS… Something like this, picking landmarks along my path to give my brain a starting and ending point to practice each of my Pilates-Walk concepts.

While there is a sequence, method, and order to the way you've learned each of the components of your healthy movement habits for a great Pilates-Walk stride, don't worry if, once you get out there and start walking, you can't remember the order in which to layer in each concept.

Yes, your body will love you and it might figure things out more quickly if you can go through the sequence in order, but you might find your brain bouncing around from your feet, to your shoulders, to your S-spot, to your abs… It's okay to let the trouble spots you notice be the next thing you focus on! With a little time and practice, you'll integrate all of these healthy movement habits into your stride for an efficient, whole-body Pilates-Walk workout.

Practice – Pilates-Walk Workout

Focus on each of the Pilates-Walk concepts during your walking workouts:

1. Begin with Breathing, Bolts, S-Spot, and Abdominals.

2. Then Pay Attention to Your Longer Stride: POS, Leg & Hip Mechanics.

3. Don't Forget Your Feet! "Heel, Ball, Toe... Away We Go!"

4. Add A Good Pendulum Arm Swing. Move the Blades & the Arms. (*Swing the whole arm not just the forearm, being sure the arms don't cross center*).

5. Breathe Deeply to Improve Posture and Lift the Ribs Up Off the Hips to Stay TALL.

6. Allow the Arm Swing to Rotate the Torso from the Belly Button Up. Oblique Abs & Spine Rotators are assisting.

You will notice that walking while you're using all these muscle groups and thinking about correctly using your Pilates-Walk concepts takes more brain-power and body work. If you feel overly-fatigued during your walking workouts from working muscles that you haven't been using, back off a bit. You can keep moving, just focus on something else and give what's getting too tired a little bit of rest.

Whatever you do, don't give it up. This brain and body work is helping to connect mind, body, and movement. First, your brain has to understand what you're doing to be able to send the right messages to your muscles. Then, you have to notice if what you've asked your body to do is happening correctly. Changing habits for better health is a process that will take time and practice to perfect.

If you know you're doing things correctly, great job! Your brain and body are working well together. If you can sense that your brain is sending the right message, but your body hasn't figured it out yet, be patient with yourself. Use the practice exercises in this book to help you re-train your body and reinforce these new movement habits. With every step you take you have the opportunity to find, feel, and fine-tune your body mechanics for better health. As your new Pilates-Walk muscle and movement patterns become stronger, you will be able to go farther and faster than ever before, and feel great with every step.

With time and practice, all of your Pilates-Walk concepts will integrate into your subconscious being. Without even thinking about what you're doing when you walk, your body will be moving efficiently, activating the right muscles, and helping you maintain a well-balanced body to stay strong, fit, flexible, and pain-free. But, until this happens...pay attention to what you're doing. When you're standing, sitting, and working to help develop your new and improved healthy movement habits.

10 Point Pilates-Walk™ Checklist

Use this 10 Point Pilates-Walk™ Checklist to help keep your brain and body connected to all the important healthy movement habits you have to practice during your walking workouts.

10 Point Pilates-Walk™ Checklist

1. Posture – On a Moving Plumb-Line
2. Breathing – Fill Back of Rib cage
3. Bolts # 1 & #2 – Lift & Support
4. S-Spot Leads
5. Sexy Hip Swing / Low Abs Smile
6. POS – Wide Stride, Legs Behind You
7. Feet – Heel, Ball, Flipper Toes
8. Maintain Core Support
9. Arm Swing – Blades and Arms
10. Spine Rotation (*from the waist up*)

You now have everything you need to get started improving your stride and enhancing your whole-body health during your walking workouts. Pay attention to your Pilates-Walk training principles during your walking workouts, and use your practice exercises to reinforce the Pilates-walk concepts as often as needed.

For the first couple of weeks, taking 10-15 minutes to go through your practice exercises before you walk will make finding everything while you're walking easier. But most importantly, get outside, enjoy the fresh air, and start putting your new and improved Pilates-Walk stride to work. Grab a friend, and have FUN walking to improve your whole-body health!

Pilates-Walk™ Practice Exercises

Use this Pilates-Walk™ Practice Exercise Checklist on the next page as a Quick Reference Guide to help you practice your preparatory Pilates-Walk exercises. These exercises will strengthen your mind-body connection and improve both support and functional mobility to enhance your gait and body mechanics for a healthy stride.

Your ultimate goal is to take the support, and healthy movement habits developed with these basic exercises, and incorporate what you're finding and feeling into your walking workouts.

You can use these practice exercises as a warm-up before you go out for a walk. Or, perhaps, take little "breaks" while you're walking to do a practice exercise, and then add that support back into your walking workout. Repeat this process throughout your walk to reinforce all the Pilates Walk concepts for a healthy stride.

Most of all, get out and enjoy the great, whole-body benefits of WALKING! Use your Pilates-Walk™ training principles to fine-tune your fitness and maximize the whole-body health benefits of your walking workouts. Plus you can continue to practice as you move throughout the day with the walking you do in everyday life. Every step you take is an opportunity to stay healthy!

Pilates-Walk™ Practice Exercises Checklist

Prep, Breathing & Support

1. Standing Posture	Alignment & Support	Throughout day
2. Scarf Breathing (w / or w/o scarf)	10-20 Breaths	Throughout day
3. Seated Bolt #1 – Pubic Bone to S-Spot	Hold 10-30 sec.	5x
4. Seated Bolt #2 – 2" below navel to back ribs	Hold 10-30 sec.	5x
5. Standing Bolt #1 & Bolt #2	Hold 10-30 sec.	5x
6. Seated "S" Spot Magnet	Hold 10-30 sec.	5x
7. Standing "S" Spot Magnet	Hold 10-30 sec.	5x
8. Low Ab Smile	Hold 5-10 sec.	5x

Low Back, Hips and Core

9. Seated Sexy Hips (Alternate Low Ab Smile)	Alternate Bolt #2, rt/left	5-10x each side
10. Standing Sexy Hips (1 Knee Bend)	Alternate Sides	5-10x each side

Posterior Oblique System - Wide Stride

11. POS – One Leg Lift Back	Standing	5-10x each side
12. Prone – One Leg Lift Back	Lying on Stomach	5-10 each side

Feet – Ankles, Arches & Toes

13. Seated Feet: Flex & Point	L-Sit	5-10x each side
14. Standing Calf Stretch to Flipper Toes	Chair or Wall	5-10x each side

More Core

15. Standing Roll Down on the Wall	Breathe Naturally	3-5x
16. Criss-Cross Abs	Breathe	8-20x

Arms, Shoulders / Spine & Rib Cage

17. Seated Arm Swing	Whole arm/spine twist	30 sec – 1 min
18. Standing Arm Swing	Whole arm/spine twist	30 sec – 1 min
19. Seated Simple Twist	Sequential rotation	5-10x alt. sides

*Note: Finish your Pilates-Walk Practice exercises with either the Standing Roll Down on the wall, or Lie on your back and Hug Both Knees to Your Chest to "center" your spine.

ABOUT THE AUTHOR:
ALIESA GEORGE, PMA-CPT

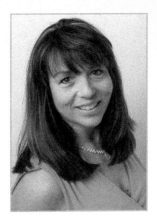

Aliesa George is the founder of Centerworks®. She is a healthy movement habits expert, author, teacher-trainer, mentor, and workshop presenter with a focus on Pilates, foot fitness, and functional movement. Aliesa has a BFA in Modern Dance, and holds certifications with PMA, and ACE. She loves problem-solving and developing safe, effective, creative programs that stay true to "working the Pilates system" while keeping challenged clients safe and healthy clients focused so that they may improve form and function, develop better whole-body health, and ultimately achieve wellness success.

Aliesa has been teaching movement for more than 30 years, and teaching Pilates for over 20 years. As a competitive gymnast and modern dancer who was plagued with chronic back and foot injuries, Aliesa, discovered Pilates when searching for a career change due to a voice injury. Pilates improved her posture and breathing habits, resolved her voice problems. Because of this, she could continue enjoying her passion for teaching, helping people stay fit, and showing them how to connect mind, body, and movement.

Aliesa has experience teaching a wide range of populations and fitness levels from dancers, athletes, runners, and tri-athletes to children, seniors, those challenged with injuries and chronic health problems, she enjoys every client who is eager to learn more about themselves from the inside out. Aliesa is the author of numerous wellness resources including Pilates exercise manuals and the books: "A Barrel of Fun," "Fantastic Feet!" and "Pulse Power." She is also the creator of the Super Ankles Foot-Fit Board Workout and the RunFit Kit, and always has new books, workshops/ webinars, and projects in development!

WALKING AND WELLNESS RESOURCES FROM CENTERWORKS®

Find the products and resources recommended at www.centerworks.com and incorporate them into your fitness routine to help improve your whole-body health and fitness and walking technique.

Posture & Breathing

Take the Quick Posture Quiz
www.centerworks.com/functional-movement/

Posture Principles for Health
www.centerworks.com/store/product/posture-principles-for-health/

Breathing Tips and Techniques
www.centerworks.com/category/functional-movement/breathing/

POS – Pilates, Core, Hip Mechanics, Healthy Shoulders, and Whole-Body Conditioning

Pilates Arc Barrel Combo

Utilize the Pilates Arc Barrel, *A Barrel of Fun!* Book and Workout Video Combo to restore proper movement, strength and flexibility of the spine, and get easy-to-follow guidelines for 45 different Arc Barrel exercises with over 200 photos in the *A Barrel of Fun!* book by Pilates expert Aliesa George.

A Barrel of Fun! (Pilates Arc Barrel Workout book)

Get the health improvement benefits of the Pilates Arc Barrel exercises to increase core strength, improve flexibility and mobility of the spine, help reduce shoulder-pain with better arm and shoulder mechanics, strengthen hips, improve gait for walking and running and help eliminate lower back pain.

Pulse-Power™ The Daily Dozen 10 Minute Workout Plan

Get ready to embrace new levels of personal power while you improve strength, flexibility, and fitness. By incorporating these easy and effective Pulse-Power exercises into your workouts, you will see rapid improvements in core support, balance, and body control.

e-Courses

Participate in these e-Courses to fine tune your Whole-Body Health and improve your Pilates-Walk™ technique. Visit Centerworks.com for these and other virtual training courses available from Centerworks.

Foam Roller Fitness Exercise Tips & Core Training Techniques

Are you ready to tap into the transformational training benefits of foam roller fitness? Discover simple ways to utilize the foam roller to enhance your workouts, get more from your core, develop strong abs and a healthy back, and maximize the whole-body health benefits from your head to your toes.

How to Effectively Engage the Pelvic Floor to Help Strengthen the Core

Gain access to the powerful health enhancing benefits of finding and using the muscles of your pelvic floor to help strengthen your core.

6-Dot Strategy for Effective Rotation of the Spine

Unleash the power of the 6-Dot Strategy to help transform the benefits of all of your Oblique core training exercises. Explore the feeling of easy, effortless movement and effective sequential rotation of the spine.

6 Simple Training Tips for Functional Movement at the Hips

Discover simple training tips and exercise strategies to help you keep your hips strong, fit, and flexible. Help improve balanced muscle development, body mechanics, and reduce or eliminate chronic back and hip pain. How we're using the muscles of our hips matter for good health and wellness success.

Foot Fitness

RunFit Foot Fitness Kit

If you walk or run and want to avoid foot pain problems like Plantar Fasciitis, ankle sprains, shin splints, foot cramps, Achilles tendon problems and more... The foot-fitness products in this Runfit Kit will be a valuable addition to your training program. For the price of one good pair of running shoes, you'll have everything you need to keep your feet fit for a lifetime of good health.

Fantastic Feet! Exercises to Strengthen the Ankles, Arches, and Toes (Book and mini foot-kit combo)

Good health starts from the ground up! This easy-to-use *Fantastic Feet!* exercise book will provide you with exercises for healthy and happy feet.

Super-Ankles Foot-Fit Board Bundle

If your sport or daily activities have you walking, running or jumping, the Super Ankle Board workout can be a super-great training tool to help keep your feet fit!

Yamuna Foot Savers

If you suffer from arch pain, foot cramps or plantar fasciitis, these plastic half-spheres are an intense, powerful tool to help you improve foot function and re-educate your feet. They help to improve gait, alignment, and muscle tone, stimulate reflexology points, strengthen arches, increase range of motion, and stimulate and elongate the muscles of the calves, thighs, hips, and lower back.

Centerworks® Acupressure Foot Massage Mat

Quickly help improve the health and fitness of your feet. By walking or "marching" on your Foot Massage Mat for a quick 2-minute (or less) workout, you can stimulate the foot reflexology points on the soles of your feet to begin releasing stress and tension and start increasing energy and vitality.

These foot care resources and more are available in the foot fitness section of the Centerworks.com store.

Movement Mentoring: Workshops, Classes, Personal Training, and Coaching

Learn it LIVE! Interested in bringing a Pilates-Walk™ workshop or other fun Pilates, foot-fitness, or healthy movement habits training program with Aliesa George to your city, studio, or club? Contact Aliesa today at www.centerworks.com and get started planning your next event NOW!

Do you feel like you need a little extra coaching to get your wellness program working? Are you struggling with chronic aches and pains and are ready for them to go away? Would you like to fine-tune your technique to improve sports performance? Contact Aliesa and inquire about special VIP Day packages, and healthy movement habit mentoring programs.

For updates on workshops, eCourses, and events with Aliesa be sure to:

Subscribe to Centerworks Wellness Success eNews
www.centerworks.com/newsletter/

Like Us on Facebook
www.Facebook.com/centerworks

Connect on Linkedin
www.Linkedin.com/in/centerworks

Follow us on Twitter
www.Twitter.com/aliesageorge

See What's Up on Pinterest
www.Pinterest.com/centerworks

Check out our YouTube Videos
www.Youtube.com/centerworks

Printed in the USA
CPSIA information can be obtained
at www.ICGtesting.com
LVHW010413160324
774593LV00002B/404